THE EARTH OF LOVE

The Earth of Love

DOMINIQUE DAVIS

Dominique Davis

Copyright © 2023 by Dominique Davis

All rights reserved. No part of this book may be reproduced in any manner whatsoever without written permission except in the case of brief quotations embodied in critical articles and reviews.

First Printing, 2023

Dedicated to my inner little girl.

CONTENTS

Root Chakra Pt. 1
1

Death Pt. 2
2

Home Pt. 2
3

Rocks And Stones Pt. 3
4

Touch Pt. 3
5

Root Chakra Pt. 2
6

Falling Pt. 2
8

Body Pt. 1
9

Gravity Pt. 3
10

Pause
11

Weighted Blanket
12

Mud Pt. 2

13

In And Back

15

Gravity Pt. 1

16

Bones Pt. 2

17

Holding On Pt. 2

19

Falling Pt. 1

21

Crystals Pt. 3

22

In And Down

23

Pause

24

Death Pt. 1

25

Crystals Pt. 1

26

Food Pt. 1

28

Touch Pt. 2

29

Bones Pt. 3

30

Food Pt. 2
31

Food Pt. 3
32

Rocks And Stones Pt. 2
34

Home Pt. 1
35

Pause
36

Holding On Pt. 3
37

Grief Pt. 2
38

Touch Pt. 1
40

Mud Pt. 3
41

Holding On Pt. 1
42

Slow Down Pt. 1
43

Home Pt. 3
44

Death Pt. 3
46

Gravity Pt. 2
47

Body Pt. 3
48

Body Pt. 2
49

Pause
50

Slow Down Pt. 2
51

Rock And Stones Pt. 1
52

Boundaries Pt. 1
53

Boundaries Pt. 2
54

Boundaries Pt. 3
55

Grief Pt. 3
56

Crystals Pt. 2
57

Bones Pt. 1
58

Mud Pt. 1
59

Grief Pt. 1
60

Apana Vayu
61

Root Chakra Pt. 3

62

Slow Down Pt. 3

63

Ayurvedic Wellness Coach

64

ROOT CHAKRA PT. 1

An anchor of red hot energy
Rivaling the pit of a volcano
Connecting me to the core of the Earth

Under the authority of the great mama
I have the right to grace this planet
Under the eyes of the gods and goddesses
I am protected and secure
Along with the Sequoia trees
My roots run deep
Along with the butterflies and the bees
All of my resources are met

And with my feet planted firmly
I rest in faith
In absolute trust
There is no one to be
But me
There is nowhere to go
But right here

I am safe

DEATH PT. 2

Every month I die
By the wisdom of my womb

She lets go in blood
She is transformed drenched in red
I rest so she can do what comes natural to her
So I can hear her whispering the secrets of the universe
So she can release what is no longer serving us

Every month I rise from the dead
By the wisdom of my womb

HOME PT. 2

I am cleaning out my home
Of all the things that were brought in without my permission,
Due to my lack of knowledge,
Because of fear
I am making space for all of the magnificence to come forth

My home will be a garden
Filled with roses
Lavender
Mugwort
Skullcap
Cinnamon
Orange peels
Blueberry scones
Coconut milk baths
Ginger foot soaks
Warm sesame oil massages

The smell of raspberries fill the air
As I make love to myself
On red silk sheets

Candles burst aflame
As I wrap myself around myself
And taste the flavors of my core

In my home
I contain everything I will ever need

ROCKS AND STONES PT. 3

When I first saw myself
Really saw myself
I cried tears that were the weight of a million stones

They tumbled down my face so slowly
As if they were savoring the feeling of their descent

They must've been waiting for this
For things that are heavy must fall
Or be put down to carry no longer

After they fell
I saw myself anew
Glistening
A lightness flowing through me

TOUCH PT. 3

After all of the roughness
After all of the hands that mishandled me

Who knew
It would be the hands that landed softly on my skin
That caused me to break open and fall apart

Who knew
It would be the hands that caressed me so gently
That caused the biggest waves to flow through me

Who knew
It would be the open palm
And not the closed fist
That allowed me to feel the most safe

I can finally blossom into a flower
Not by the hand that picks me from the ground
But by the hand that simply turns me towards their face
And uses their senses to delight in me

ROOT CHAKRA PT. 2

Gently close your eyes
Envision a glowing red ball the color of fresh blood
Resting at the base of your pelvis

Breathe in
The ball expands
Breathe out
It melts down your thighs
Like the red icee running down your chin as a little kid

Breathe in
The ball expands
Breathe out
The ball liquifies and pours down your legs
Like lava running down Mt. Vesuvius

Breathe in
The ball expands
Breathe out
The glowing red ball travels down your thighs
Down your calves
Through your feet
Into the Earth
Making a path straight to the core

   Your red hot energy is now mingling with the energy of the Great Mama
      Swirling around
      Bouncing off of one another

Smiling and laughing together

You've found your connection to the Source
Whenever you feel alone or lost
Guide yourself down this path

FALLING PT. 2

If you're going to fall
Fall like the petals of a flower
Letting go when the time is just right

Landing on the soil
Gently meeting its demise
Trusting in it's disintegration

Becoming one with the Earth
Knowing that death does not exist
It will only return to source

And transform
What was once a rose
Will now be a peony
Or maybe a daisy for bees to graze
Or maybe grass for caterpillars to munch

Be like the petal of a flower
Simply grateful to be a part of the circle of life
Flowing where it wishes

BODY PT. 1

This body
Was made for pleasure

I was made for honey to dance with my tongue
I was made for roses to be placed under my nose
I was made for the sound of ocean waves to fall upon my ears
I was made for silk sheets to graze against my skin
I was made to witness the magnificence of the mountains and the sky

As I indulge in the wonders of my senses
Mother Earth sends her unending love

GRAVITY PT. 3

You are a dichotomy
Not only do you make me feel like I am floating on clouds
You also make me feel like I am sinking into the Earth

A new kind of gravity
Where I'm suspended in time
My heart is flying with the eagles
And my hips are swimming with the koi fish

A grounded expansion
An ascended death

PAUSE

*Take this moment to stop and look around you.
Soaking in where you are right now.
You are where you are for a reason.
What lesson are you meant to be learning?*

WEIGHTED BLANKET

No longer will sleep elude me
No longer will my racing mind awaken me
No longer will tension keep me safe

I've given myself permission to let go
To melt
To fall into the support of the mattress underneath me
To be held down
As if gravity became my newfound lover

This body is so used to running away
Finally, I get to stay put
So rest can catch up to me

MUD PT. 2

I remember the first time I traveled into my root
What was supposed to be plush and glowing reds and oranges
Was a muddy cave

I saw darkness
I felt cold
I heard screams

There was a dark woman there
Dressed in black
Hair flowing to the ground

She was holding the hand of a beast
An extraordinary creature of skin and bones
They opened their arms out to me

Against my own will I went to them
I found my breath and they breathed with me
"Thank you for seeing us" they said

And suddenly they disappeared
And I returned to this dimension
Feeling like I was covered in mud from head to toe
I knew they were standing right beside me

So I ran a bath
And together we cleansed ourselves
And all of a sudden
I felt a sudden warmth become alive in my womb

I will forever praise the mud
That the dark woman and the beast
Made home

IN AND BACK

Breathe in
Allow your breath to fill your belly
And then rise and fill up your chest

Hold it for a second
Feel into the expansion of your body

Breathe out
And now
Imagine your breath leaving your body through the back of your heart

Drop your shoulders
Relax your chest
Sigh it out

Bring all of your awareness to your back body
Your place of unwavering trust and unending support
Your place of receiving

Breathe deeply
Filling up your entire torso

Hold

Exhale slowly
And like angel wings
Let your breath unfurl behind you

GRAVITY PT. 1

The universe adores me so much
That gravity was put in place
So I could always be planted on the Earth
Securely connected to the ultimate life force
Where joy is of infinite supply
Where love is ever present

BONES PT. 2

My world is in between my hips
A world unlike any other
Where rivers of blood flow
Where mountains of bone grow

The night sky is full of stars
The day sky is full of dandelions
Bridges made of books
On the highest hill, my thrones of thorns

When I dance, tornadoes form
Thunder claps for me
Pleasure pours from above
Watering me, drenching me in ecstasy

The dandelions drink up,
The lotus flowers blossom
Creation in constant motion

When I want to rest,
Butterflies carry me to fields of wheat
The smell of fresh baked bread
My lullaby

Red cardinals bring my cinnamon tea
When I awake
I meditate and hum along with the beehives
Letting the honeybees give me kisses

My breasts reach for the sky
My Yoni is connected to the roots of the trees

In my world between my thighs
I am the door
I am the portal

The only way in is through me
The only way out is through me

HOLDING ON PT. 2

Shoulders pushed up by my ears
Stomach sucked in
Tailbone tucked under

Chest caved in
Arms glued to my side
Stuck
Tension ruling me

I had nothing to hold me
So the only safety I knew
Was trying to curl into myself
Trying to hide

I curled so deep inside of myself
I reached my core
And heard my Great Mother tell me
"Unfurl my love
Trust in your rebirth"

Ever so slowly
I let go

Dropping my shoulders
Sticking out my tail
Letting my breath expand my belly
Opening my heart to receive
Lifting my hands to the sky

This freedom
This breaking open
Hurts so good

FALLING PT. 1

When I am with you
I fall so deep
I descend into myself

And I find you swimming in my waters
And together
We fall to the ocean floor
Swallowed by the sand
Landing into darkness

All we feel is each other
All we hear are our hearts beating
All we want is more
I can't hold enough of you
You can't taste enough of me
How much deeper can we go?

So deep, we find stars
The moon greets us
And we howl back like the wild wolves we are
Your fingertips caressing me
My lips grazing you
We rest in the moonlight

Alas, we start to see the sun rise into the night sky
How beautiful
We fell so deep, the light found us

CRYSTALS PT. 3

Everyday
I visit the graveyard of myself
Digging for power that's been buried alive

I wear a belt of black tourmaline
I must not fear the dark bloody depths for I came from them
A garland of bloodstone
I will sing the songs of the dead and they will hear me clearly
An amethyst tiara
I am protected as I encounter my demons

If you see me
Eyes wide from seeing ghosts
Picking mud from underneath my fingernails
Know that I've just come back from the underworld
And I've returned with hidden treasures

IN AND DOWN

Breathe in through your nose
Exhale
Let your breath roll down your legs
For the force that lives in your hips
Your thighs
Your knees
Your calves
Your ankles
Your feet
Is a grounding force
A connecting force

Keep your attention
On the soles of your feet
There is a incomprehensible intelligence
In acknowledging
Where you are standing
For you have been placed there
For magical reasons

Be still
Listen
To the wisdom of here and now
Be still
Feel
The expansiveness of the present moment

PAUSE

Take this moment to give a bit of gratitude to yourself.
What do you absolutely love about yourself?
And what about the thing that you absolutely hate...
Do you have it within you to show it a little bit of love?

DEATH PT. 1

Breaking apart my foundation
Revealing rot
Decaying matter
The stench of old

I didn't know what to make of this death
I first thought it would be best to turn away
To ignore the dying matter of myself

But
Deep down I knew
There is wisdom in the deterioration
This decay is the essence of change

And I am an alchemist
Armed with love and compassion
Awareness is my sword
Faith is my shield

So I show up fully present
I bring marigolds
I sing the hymns of the Apache warrior
Honoring the beauty of dying

For what rots
Will be witnessed with such a softness
That it will lace the cocoon of a caterpillar
And return to me on the wings of a butterfly

CRYSTALS PT. 1

I lie on my back
And adorn myself with the jewels of the Earth

Rubies between my thighs
Connecting me to Gaia's fierce love
Anchored in her unwavering strength

Citrine placed on my pelvis
I am the infinite flow
For my very existence is the love making of gods and goddesses

Sunstone right above my belly button
Igniting the thousand suns that burn in my belly
A woman born from a blazing fire

Emerald resting between my breasts
My heart is the greatest forcefield
Drawing in blessings from every direction

A necklace of Aquamarine
Carrying the vibrations of my voice to the most distant stars
I am heard in every corner of the sky

Sodalite over my third eye
To not just look
But to see

A crown of Moonstone
For the clearest aura

My sensitivity is my superpower

What magic is it
To have this Earthly body
And this body of Light

FOOD PT. 1

A person who never got the chance
To breath into the life of their belly
Sucked in as to not take up space
Breath being held because existence isn't safe
There's nothing there
So food becomes the source of feeling

Only when stuffed to the brim
Will safety ensue
Only when bursting at the seams
Will the body feel alive

With the utmost courage
I've broken the cycle

Now, I place my hand on my belly
I feel it rise and fall with my breath
And I ask myself?

Is my body hungry for food?
Or is it my spirit that's hungry for something more?

TOUCH PT. 2

You touch me with a fascination
With a sense of awe
And also a sense of relief

Finally

*"The woman that fits into the palms of my hands
Has arrived"*

BONES PT. 3

A glorious creature
Of skin and bones
Lives in my shadows

She is ravished
Blinded with hunger
Mad with longing

She wants to take and take and take
And take and take
To fulfill her yearning

She only knows how to devour

I have been tasked with allowing this beautiful beast
To sit with me at meal time
And show her the pleasure of using every sense
To savor every smell, every taste
Every sound, every sight,
Every single feeling

My heart is big enough
To hold space for her
As she stumbles over herself
As she screams out all of the pain

The Earth is big enough
To hold both of us

FOOD PT. 2

Enter your kitchen
The heart of the home

Feel your feet pressing firmly into the cool tiles
Sturdy countertops holding bowls and plates

Hear the water running down the drain
Filling containers and taking their shape

Feel the warmth of the fire heating up pans
Melting coconut oil and ghee

Smell the fragrances filling the air
Making your mouth water

Breathe into the space in your belly
Patiently waiting to be filled with nourishment

A grounded body
With senses lit up
Is a healthy body
A body that can take in food
Transmute it into the necessary nutrients
Excrete the waste
And become the life that it has taken in

FOOD PT. 3

Honey
Basmati rice
Blueberry muffins
Sweet potatoes
Licorice root
Sweet

Lemons
Sauerkraut
Tamarind
Grapefruit
Kombucha
Sour

Miso paste
Soy sauce
Olives
Salt fish
Tamari
Salty

Ginger
Cayenne pepper
Jalapeño
Mustard seeds
Wasabi
Pungent

Kale

Aloe Vera
Dandelion root
Cacao
Bitter

Cranberries
Chickpeas
Green bananas
Pomegranate
Astringent

ROCKS AND STONES PT. 2

Ever since I was a little girl
Everytime I went to a new place

I scoured the ground
Looking for a stone

A stone that spoke to my heart
A piece of the Earth that wanted to belong to me

Feeling the weight of it in my pocket
It was a gentle reminder
That no matter where I am

I am connected to something bigger
I am home always

HOME PT. 1

When the desire to escape ceases
That's when you know
You are home

When you've found the place you want to run back to, clutching good news in your arms
When you've found the place that you want to decorate with the tulips you've just picked in the meadow
When you've found the place you want to open all the curtains and let light reach all the corners
You are home

In the bed where the covers feel like the arms of God
On the floor that holds your body and catches your tears
Behind the door in the room where the walls echo back your screams
You are not alone

In this home where everything is alive
The cluttered closets holding the mess of the past
The empty spaces buzzing with new possibilities
The dust flying up as you walk by
The silence surrounding you
The little noises that happen even when nothing else is moving
Like the house is breathing

When you have the desire to exhale and fully let go
That's when you know
You are home

PAUSE

Stop.
Kiss each shoulder.
Kiss the back of each hand.
Softly rub your thighs.
You are here.
You are beautiful.

HOLDING ON PT. 3

On days like this
When my strength looks like breaking down
I have no desire to hold on
I have no energy to keep myself together

So I fall apart into pieces
And I hope
That there will be something to break my fall

GRIEF PT. 2

The girl I once was
No longer serves me

She is meek
Voiceless
Frozen in time

And even though I know I must let her go
It still hurts
She is apart of me
She is the reason I am right here in this present moment

In all of her defenses
In all of her shortcomings
In all of her fears
She persevered

And it is with the utmost reverence
That I praise her
For her infinite strength
Her incomprehensible wisdom
Her inner spark that she knew she must cover to protect
I praise her
For her hiding away
Her playing dead
Her numbing of herself
I praise her
For she worked with what she had
She did the best she could

And she is ready to return to the void
She is exhausted

The girl I once was
No longer serves me
So I grieve her

And with an open heart
I leave a trail of roses
For her exit

TOUCH PT. 1

My skin craves loving hands
That know when to hold
And when to let go

Reading my goosebumps like braille
Kneading my scars into a soft dough
Exploring the playground of my curves
Feeling into the depth of my valleys

My skin is thirsty for fingers
That run across me like I am a piano
Making a song out of me
Digging into me
Striking cords that were never before played

My body longs to melt
In the palms of one that has no fear of fluidity
Hands that want to become an expert
At holding new shapes

MUD PT. 3

You must get familiar with getting dirty
You must come to love the mud

For there is no better offering
To the gods and goddesses
Than your mud dipped heart

It lets them know that you had the courage
To dig
And meet the mess

It lets them know that you had the strength
To carry that mess
And place it at their altar

There is no shame
In calling on bigger forces
To aid in your alchemy

They will take your mud
And swallow it to the depths of their bellies
Where they can digest it by the strongest fires
And assimilate the nutrients

Unto you they will return the hidden gold

HOLDING ON PT. 1

What a great gift
To be able to hold on to beautiful things

With my arms
I hold on to my lover
I hold on to a bouquet of daffodils

With my womb
I hold on to the resilient stories of my mother
I hold on to magic of the Cosmos

With my hands
I hold on to a pen that bleeds the anguish of my heart
I hold on to Rumi's words

And with my heart
I hold on to all of the love thats comes and goes
I hold on to all of the softness

SLOW DOWN PT. 1

Slow down, you reminded me
Stay still for a second
And feel it pulsating inside of you
Just breathe, baby
I got you

As I finally entered my body and left my mind behind
You were all I could feel
In that moment, we were the entire world
And the rivers inside of me started to rise
I could feel every tingle, every spark

I've never felt so alive

HOME PT. 3

I always had the urge to run away
I remember always feeling like I was never home
Like there was no place on the Earth for me

The only home I had to escape to was my mind
But how volatile is that?
Thoughts bouncing off my skull
Flying at 90 mph
No rest in sight

I could not live there
And I was determined to find a place for me
I no longer had the energy to keep running

So I looked to a place that was always there
The place that never left
Even through all the hatred
All the abuse
All the mindless numbing

My body

And how glorious?
As soon as I opened the door
The sensations came pouring through
Waves of shivers
Bursting tears
Unlocked screams
Jumping for joy

She was waiting for me
Trusting in my return
No resentment for my having left
I was welcomed with opened arms

Never again
Will I abandon my home
My safe haven
Where I need for nothing
And everything I want is already mine

DEATH PT. 3

I heard somewhere that life belongs to death

That we can only taste the sweetness of life
When death is near

That we can only see clearly
When we are looking through death's eyes

That our hearts can only open to receive
When we make offerings to death

I always looked to life for my lessons
Maybe death can be my teacher too

GRAVITY PT. 2

My great mother knew
Of the capacity of my mind
To soar great distances
To travel to unknown destinations
To make a mess of situations
To be in thirteen different places at once

My great mother knew
That there needed to be a force greater than any other
That presses me down
Holds me together
Keeps things in order
Stops my thoughts from flying away

Whenever I am feeling alone
And the lover inside of me is too tired
I feel into the gravity around me
It's invisible arms pressing into me

I am held always

BODY PT. 3

The beauty of the mountains rests in my teeth and bones
The fluidity of water flows in my blood and tears
The spark of flames lives in my core and my beating heart
The grace of the wind moves in my lungs
And this body takes up it's rightful space

I was made in the image of the Earth
She is my mother
I am her beloved child
I will praise her creation
I will revere her masterpiece

BODY PT. 2

In a world where it's normal for the mind to run the show
I return to my body

Where magic lies dormant
Where my intuition and I speak our own language
Where my desires are alive inside my beating heart
Where my internal compass guides me
Where I heal with every deep breath

I am grateful for the logical nature of my mind
Helping me solve problems
Allowing proper judgment

At the same time

It's my body's innate intelligence that carries me
It's the instant spark of inspiration that flickers in my belly
It's the flood of chills that says *"Yes please, keep doing that"*
It's through my relaxed muscles that my prana flows

The ultimate creator
Has made me in such a way
That if I stop and listen
If I stop and feel into myself
I shall know the path to take

PAUSE

There is a piece of love around you at this very moment.
Find it.
Hold it close.

SLOW DOWN PT. 2

I had found safety in speed
Walking quickly so no one could catch me
Talking quickly so no one would interrupt me
Acting quickly so I wouldn't have to feel doubt
Always thinking of the future so I didn't have to feel the present moment

I learned that you can only move so quickly
Before you run out of gas
Before you burn out

ROCK AND STONES PT. 1

Sometimes
I don't feel strong enough to carry my grief
Weighing heavy on my chest like a thousand rocks
Sitting in my throat like a million stones

Stop resisting my love
Stop trying to lift the rocks and stones
Let them rest there

Feel yourself sinking under the pressure of them
No judgment
Send them love
And they will begin to erode

By the winds of my breath
By the steady dropping of my tears
They crumble
They become lighter and lighter

And I am in awe
Of how my softness can move mountains

BOUNDARIES PT. 1

I was violated before I could even speak
Which led me to believe
That my being was at the dispense of the world around me

I held the door open for others
As they came in
Wreaked havoc
And left
Without a please or thank you

I was not mine

BOUNDARIES PT. 2

I decided
I had been taken from enough
No fucking more

So I erected stone walls
I built dams
I put up guards
Electrical fences
Spike strips
Mine fields

I shut the door
I turned off the lights
Now nothing can come in
And nothing can come out

BOUNDARIES PT. 3

Kali Ma found her way into my heart
She told me her secrets
And showed me her biggest fears

But she told me I must not back down
I mustn't let my heart become cold
It's time to step from behind the walls with faith and conviction

Every day
She carries her fear
And throws it into the fire of love
And around it she dances

Eyes glowing red
A necklace of skulls
Swaying hips fashioned with a skirt of arms who reached without permission

She hands me her sword
And tells me
"Yield it fiercely
And gracefully hold the head of the offender up for everyone to see

You are a powerful woman
Armed with the power to protect yourself
So lead with an open heart
Embrace death
And you will be shown the abundance of life"

GRIEF PT. 3

A growing life
Snatched from my womb

I knew it had to be done
Even though I daydreamed of holding you
I was not ready for you
So I made one of the hardest decisions of my life

My spirit baby
You are my angel
Watching over me
Offering guidance
Sending blessings

When sadness creeps in
And grief spills out of me
I imagine that I am being held by your consciousness

You were once a part of me
And now you are in the heavens
That must mean
There's a chance for me too

CRYSTALS PT. 2

I had given away my power
I was left empty
No fight left

My only option was to find my voice
And call it back to me

With tigers eye clutched tightly in my hands
I roared
I growled

My strength clawed it's way out of me
And I learned
That I never gave it away

I just hid it deep deep within myself
Covered and protected
And it waited
For me to seek it out again

BONES PT. 1

All the unshouted screams
All the unsung songs
All the stuffed down tears
All the unfulfilled wishes
Of all the women who came before me
Now lives in my bones

Placed there with the deepest faith
They knew I would come
They are standing behind me
Massaging my shoulder blades
Pressing into my sacrum
Urging me forward

Whenever I feel weak
Whenever I feel lost
They guide me deep inside of myself
My bones are their graveyard

I sit with them
I build a fire
They sing me to sleep
And when I wake
They send me off with a torch to light the way

Reminding me that whenever I need guidance
Come back to my bones
And listen for their whispers

MUD PT. 1

I will return to the dirt
And as I cry
The dirt will turn to mud
And I will sit in the mess

Inhaling the smell of fresh Earth
Exhaling tension
For this is the beginning

This is where life starts
This is where seeds are planted
This is where mother nature nurtures
And breaths her breath of life
This is where father sky rains down
And allows his sun to shine

In the mud, I can rest
I can sleep
Soon will be my time when I feel the air on my face

But for now
I am buried
Embracing the darkness

GRIEF PT. 1

I die over and over and over
And over
Grief has become my closest friend

I dare even say lover
Because I've learned that love is also an act of letting go
Of allowing death to visit

So the fields can be cleared
And the soil could be plowed
And new seeds can be planted

My tears will water the grounds
My screams will move the clouds so the sun can shine down

From my grief
A garden will bloom

APANA VAYU

Little Dominique
Did not have a safe place to express her big feelings
So whenever she was overcome with sadness or anger or fear
She would lay down and curl up into a little ball
Holding those big feelings inside of her tiny body
This was the only safe place for them

But I am here now
And I am aware of the magic of my being
I am aware of the downward winds
That moves down my legs
And into the Earth

My Great Mother knew
That sometimes things would feel just a bit too unbearable
So instead of curling up
I stand up
And move my body
I shake
I bounce up and down
I stomp
I wiggle
And all of the sticky stuff falls out of me
Down into the Earth
Where my Great Mother swallows it
And returns it to the void

And little Dominique and I just dance and laugh
Overcome with joy

ROOT CHAKRA PT. 3

I have a right to be here
It is safe for me to take up space
I am worthy of having my needs met

I have a right to be here
It is safe for me to be in the present moment
I am worthy of safety and security

I have a right to be here
It is safe for me to trust myself
I am worthy of belonging and acceptance

I have a right to be here
It is safe for me to nourish myself
I am worthy of calmness and peace

I have a right to be here
It is safe for me to simply be
I am worthy of love just because

SLOW DOWN PT. 3

I realized
I find myself chasing peace
When peace finds itself running after me
Trying to catch up
Begging me to slow down
To stop
Be still
Hold my arms open
So she can crash into me

I realized
I don't need to go finding peace
I need to quit searching
And let her find me
Only, she's never lost me
She knows exactly where I am at all times
Rest assured

AYURVEDIC WELLNESS COACH

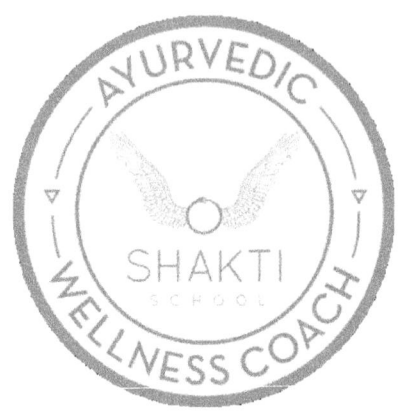

If you want to learn more about the medicine of Ayurveda and are interested in incorporating some routines into your daily life that work with your own personal constitution, I would be honored to help you get started! Reach out to me with any questions you have @theearth.ofloveayurveda@gmail.com!

Expressing the deepest gratitude for you taking the time to read these words that I have poured my love into. I wish that you have been moved to your core, that something in your spirit has been stirred, that something inside of you has been unlocked.

Printed in the USA
CPSIA information can be obtained
at www.ICGtesting.com
LVHW050233310723
753623LV00018B/1140

9 781088 179185